The
Diggum Uppers
Grave Robbing and Body Snatching in the Black Country

The Diggum Uppers:
Body-Snatching and Grave-Robbing in the Black Country

Published by
Bows, Blades and Battles Press
202 Ashenhurst Road,
Dudley,
West Midlands,
Dy1 2hz.

ISBN 978-0-9571377-3-8

First published 2017

http://bowsbladesandbattles.tripod.com

Two men placing the shrouded corpse which they have
just disinterred into a sack while Death, as a
nightwatchman holding a lantern, grabs one of the grave-
robbers from behind. Coloured drawing by T.
Rowlandson, 1775. (Wellcome Library London)

For Amelia Caitlin Rose

ABOUT THE AUTHOR

Kevin Goodman is a historian, independent researcher, writer, historical interpreter and reenactor who specializes in the history of medicine and surgery. When not appearing around the country at various historical events demonstrating aspects of medicine and surgery throughout history, he is continually being outfoxed by his young daughter.

More details can be found at:
http://bowsbladesandbattles.tripod.com

By the same author:
Ouch! A History of Arrow Wound Treatment from Prehistory to the Nineteenth Century (2012)
ISBN 978-0-9571377-0-7

The Lords of Dudley Castle and the Welsh Wars of Edward I (2014)
ISBN 978-0-9571377-1-4

Quacks and Cures: Quack Doctors and Folk Healing of the Black Country (2017)
ISBN 978-0-9571377-2-1

All are published by Bows, Blades & Battles Press

CONTENTS

ACKNOWLEDGMENTS

Many thanks to Luke Craddock–Bennett for a copy of his article 'Providence Chapel and burial ground, Sandwell, West Bromwich' which set me off on an exploration of the activities of the resurrectionists in the Black Country

Picture Acknowledgements

Page 4: William Hunter. Stipple engraving by J. Thomson, 1847, after R. E. Pine. Wellcome Library, London.

Page 5: John Hunter. Line engraving by W. Sharp, 1788, after Sir J. Reynolds, 1786. Wellcome Library, London.

Page 6: Portrait of Sir Astley Paston Cooper, bust facing left. Stipple and line engraving 20th January 1824 by L. Alais. Wellcome Library, London

Page 8: Dissection from Johannes Ketham Fasiculo de medicina (1491) Wellcome Library, London.

Page 9: Vesalius. De humani corporis fabrica libri septem ("On the fabric of the human body in seven books") (1543)

Page 24: William Sands Cox by T.H. Maguire (1854). Wellcome Library, London. Wellcome Library, London.

Page 36: Mortsafe at Oyne, Aberdeenshire. Wellcome Library, London.

Page 37: Mortsafes in Cluny graveyard, Aberdeenshire. Wellcome Library, London.

i

Not A Trap Was Heard
(Anonymous Ballad c.1820).

NOT a trap was heard, or a Charley's note
As our course to the churchyard we hurried,
Not a pigman discharg'd a pistol shot
As a corpse from the grave we unburied.
We nibbled it slily at dead of night,
The sod with our pick-axes turning,
By the nosing moonbeam's chaffing light,
And our lanterns so queerly burning.
By the noosing, &c

Few and short were the words we said,
And we felt not a bit of sorrow,
But we rubb'd with rouge the face of the dead
And we thought of the spoil for to-morrow.
The useless shroud we tore from his breast
And then in regimentals bound him,
And he looked like a swaddy taking his rest,
With his lobster togs around him.
And he looked , &c

We thought as we fill'd up his narrow bed,
Our snatching trick now no look sees ;
But the bulk and the sexton will find him fled,
And we far away towards Brooks's.
Largely they'll cheek 'bout the body that's gone
And poor Doctor Brooks they'l upbraid him ;
But nothing we care if they leave him alone
In a place where a snatcher has laid him.
But nothing we care, &c

But half of our snatching job was o'er,
When a pal tipt the sign quick for shuffling,
And we heard by the distant hoarse Charley's roar
That the beaks would be 'mongst us soon scuffling.
Slily and slowly we laid him down,
In our cart famed for snatching in story ;
Nicely and neatly we done 'em brown,
For we bolted away in our glory.
Nicely and neatly, &c

Introduction

When we imagine body snatchers or grave robbers images are conjured of foggy, moonless nights in Edinburgh or London through which dishevelled rodent-featured men push wooden handcarts along cobbled back streets, the cargo not long dead or not long exhumed….

Never do we think of it happening anywhere else, especially in the Black Country. Yet in January 2013 archaeologists excavating the site of the former nineteenth century Providence Baptist Chapel and graveyard in Sandwell Road, West Bromwich, (founded 1810), discovered evidence of the attempts which were made to prevent corpses being taken by the snatchers. One in particular was an iron structure known as a *mortsafe*, designed to prevent the body being exhumed (Craddock-Bennett 2013).

But moving the gothic imaginings aside, what were the reasons for, and the reality behind, grave robbing and body snatching in the Black Country?

Author's Note

The name" the Black Country" for this industrial area of the Westy Midlands comes from Elihu Burritt's book *Walks in the Black Country and its Green Borderland* (1868), (Burit was the American Consular Agent to Birmingham), in which he described the view of the Black Country from the top of Dudley

Castle:

"A writer of a military turn of fancy might say that it was the sublimest battle-scene ever enacted on earth . . . There was an embattled amphitheatre of twenty miles span ridged to the purple clouds. Planted at artillery intervals on this encircling ridge, and at musket-shot spaces in the dark valley between, a thousand batteries, mounted with huge ordnance, white at the mouth with the fury of the bombardment, were pouring their cross-fires of shot and shell into the cloud-works of the lower heavens. Wolverhampton, on the extreme left, stood by her black mortars which shot their red volleys into the night. Coseley and Bilston and Wednesbury replied bomb for bomb, and set the clouds on fire above with their lighted matches. Dudley, Oldbury, Albion, and Smethwick, on the right, plied their heavy breachers at the iron-works on the other side; while West Bromwich and distant Walsall showed that their men were standing as bravely to their guns, and that their guns were charged to the muzzle with the grape and canister of the mine. The canals twisting and crossing through the field of battle, showed by patches in the light like bleeding veins."

For readers who don't originate from the Black Country, the official Black Country History website[1]

---

[1] *http://blackcountryhistory.org/places*

states that the Black Country is comprised of Dudley, Walsall, Sandwell and Wolverhampton and points out: *"It has no agreed borders and no two Black Country men or women will agree on where its starts or ends"*. Just to complicate matters, my account of nefarious goings on in the churchyards and cemeteries of the Black Country will occasionally lead to a wandering across the borders into other parts of the Midlands, (but it's worth it).

1) MEDICAL DEMAND

Today, dissection is regarded as a necessary part of the training of physicians and surgeons and as a means to advance medical science. A number of surgeons who made vast contributions to medical science are known to have traded with, and even been dependent upon, resurrectionists. For example: William Hunter (1718-1783) famous for his studies on bone and cartilage; John Hunter (1728-1793) who helped to improve understanding of human teeth, bone growth and remodeling, inflammation, gunshot wounds, venereal diseases, digestion, child development, the separateness of maternal and foetal blood supplies and the role of the lymphatic system (Moore 2006) and Sir Astley Paston Cooper (1768-1841) who contributed to the understanding of ontology, vascular surgery, anatomy and pathology of the mammary glands and testicles and the pathology and surgery of hernias (Burch 2007).

The dissection of human cadavers was first practiced by the Greek physicians Herophilos (c330 to c260 B.C.) and Erasistratos (c310- c250 B.C.) at the School of Anatomy in Alexandria. Forbidden in the Roman world, the physician and surgeon Galen (129AD-200 AD) was forced to dissect Barbary apes and pigs, yet despite this, his conclusions remained uncontested until the sixteenth century when the anatomist Andreas Vesalius (1514-1564) published his *De humani corporis fabrica libri septem* (*"On the fabric of the*

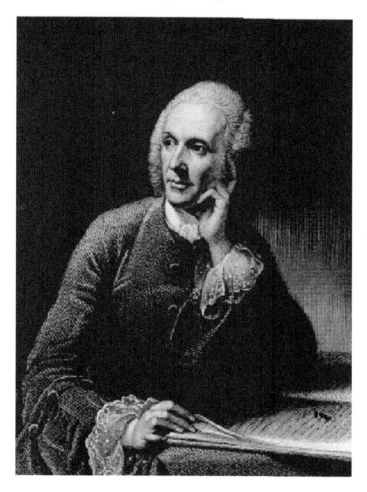

William Hunter (1718-1783) (Wellcome)

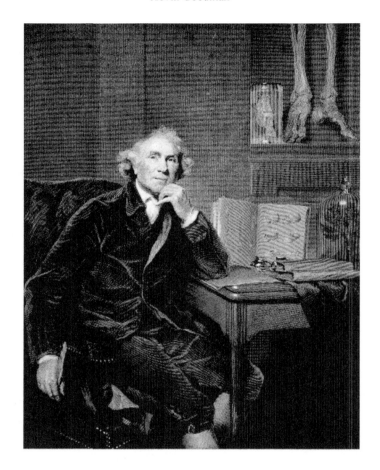

John Hunter (1728-1793) (Wellcome)

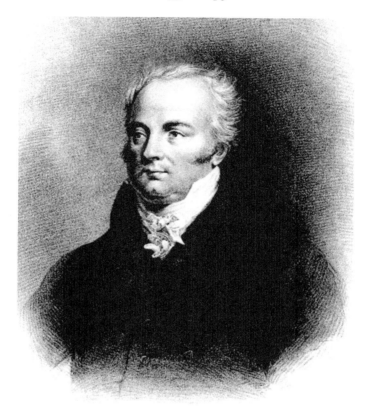

Sir Astley Paston Cooper (1768-1841) (Wellcome)

human body in seven books") in 1543. In the Christian
and early Islamic worlds the practice of cadaver
dissection was forbidden but was introduced into the
study of anatomy at the University of Bologna, circa
1300. However, it remained prohibited in England
until the sixteenth century (Quigley 2012).

As medicine and surgery became an accepted
profession the demand for human cadavers grew. It
became customary in most countries for officials to
donate the bodies of executed criminals to the
universities and medical schools. The first provision
for the supply of cadavers for anatomical dissection in
Britain was contained in the *"Seal of Cause to the Barbers
and Surgeons of Edinburgh"*, granted by the Town
Council on 1st July, 1505, and ratified by James IV
the following year. With this, physicians and surgeons
were granted the right to the cadaver of an executed
criminal once a year so they could teach, provided
they did penance for the dead man's soul. In England,
such permission was not granted until 1540 when the
Company of Barbers of London united with the
Fraternity of Surgeons to form the United Company
of Barber-Surgeons. In the Charter given by Henry
VIII provision for the study of anatomy was made as
follows:

*"the sayd maysters or governours of the mistery and
comminaltie of barbours and surgeons of London, and their
successours yerely for ever after their said discrecions at their free
liberte and pleasure shal and maie have and take without
contradiction foure persons condempned adiudged and put to*

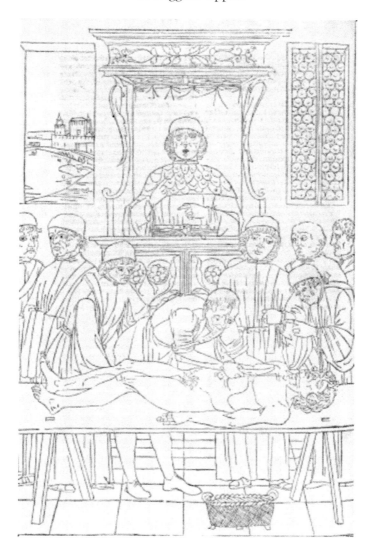

Dissection
Johannes de Ketham Fasiculo de medicina (1491) (Wellome)

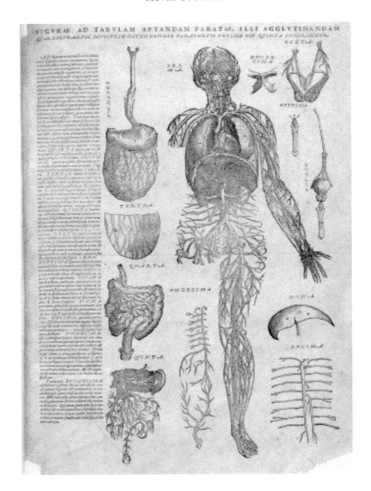

Vesalius.
From:
De humani corporis fabrica libri septem (1543)
("On the fabric of the human body in seven books")
(Wellcome)

death for feloni by the due order of the Kynges lawe of thys realme for anatomies without any further sute or labour to be made to the kynges highnes his heyres or successours for the same. And to make incision of the same deade bodies or otherwyse to order the same after their said discrecions at their pleasure for their further and better knowlage instruction insight learning and experience in the sayd scyence or facultie or surgery" (p.588, Young 1890).

In 1565, Elizabeth I granted the Royal College of Physicians four cadavers annually for dissection and Charles II increased Henry's original grant to the Barber Surgeons to six in 1663 (Quigley 2012).

By the eighteenth century the power of the monopolies of the Company of Barber-Surgeons and the Royal College of Physicians was waning. The great London hospitals of St. Thomas and St.Bartholomew were teaching anatomy and private schools run by former hospital lecturers soon appeared. The demand for anatomical subjects was growing. As part of the 1752 Murder Act under George II, common law provision was made for the statuary dissection of murderers, to add: *"...terror and peculiar infamy...to the punishment of death"* and to *"impress a just horror in the mind of the offender, and on the minds of such as shall be present, of the heinous crime of murder"*.

Black Country murderers who were dissected include William Hawkeswood of Pedmore, near Stourbridge, who was hanged for the murder of Mr. Parker in 1808 and Abel Hill who drowned his common law wife Mary Martin and their two year old son, Thomas, in a Bilston canal in February 1820. He was hung on 27th July at Stafford and his body publically dissected by the surgeon Edward Best at Workhouse Fold, Bilston. Hill's skeleton was preserved by Dr. Tom Dickenson of Bilston High Street who had a somewhat macabre sense of humour: he wired up the skeleton in a cupboard in his practice room, so that when anyone opened the cupboard door the arms of the exhibit would move forward and embrace them.

By 1760, it had become customary in the anatomical schools for students to dissect for themselves. It was also mandatory for those applying for licenses from the Royal College of Surgeons, (the successor to the Barber-Surgeons Company), to attend two full courses of anatomy with dissection. Practicing surgeons also liked to operate at least once on a cadaver before approaching a difficult case, (Hurren 2011; Wise 2004)

The demand for anatomical material escalated.

In 1793 there were over two hundred medical students in London and over a thousand by 1823. Each student required three bodies during his sixteen months of training: two for learning anatomy and one on which to practice operating techniques. The supply of convicted murderers was insufficient. The surgeons and the students were competing for less than a hundred cadavers legally available each year. And the number of legal cadavers was diminishing: in 1805 sixty eight people were executed in England and

Wales, by 1831 this had dropped to fifty two as the punishment of deportation became more common (Hurren 2011; Wise 2004).

2) THE RISE OF THE RESURRECTIONISTS

At first, the grave-robbers were amateurs, usually medical students or hospital porters who stole for their own use or their professor's. For example, an anatomy professor in Dublin, on hearing of the death of a giant named Cornelius Magrath in 1760, told his class:

"Gentlemen, I have been told that some of you in your zeal have contemplated carrying off the body. I earnestly beg you not to think of such a thing: but if you should be so carried away with your desire for knowledge that thus against my expressed wish you persist in doing so, I would have you remember that if you take only the body, there is no law whereby you can be touched, but if you so much as take a rag or a stocking with it, it is a hanging matter" (Frank 1976 p.405).

The students managed to steal Magrath's corpse from his own wake, leaving behind his clothes and shroud, and soon had him completely dissected.

A peculiarity of English law at this time was that to steal a shroud, a coffin or a corpse's clothing was considered a crime against the property of a dead person's heirs and subject to stiff punishment (including hanging). However, a person did not own their own body: it could not be willed as property; therefore, the theft of a corpse was not considered a felony, only a misdemeanour - unlawful disinterment - for which the punishment was either a fine or six months imprisonment (Hurren 2011; Wise 2004).

When the corpse of a pauper buried at Wolverhampton was stolen, the parish overseers of Willenhall, (the parish to which the pauper had belonged), who had paid for the funeral were determined to get some of their money back. The vacated coffin was subsequently offered for sale in a shop *(The Birmingham Journal* 2nd February 1828).

While body-snatching by medical students, and their professors, continued throughout the eighteenth and early nineteenth centuries there was an increase in a class of men known as *"resurrectionists"*[2] who made their living by exhuming corpses and selling them to the medical schools for dissection. At first these men were mostly cemetery watchmen, aided by a few independent desperadoes. By the early nineteenth century, however, several well-organized gangs of grave robbers had appeared in London and other large cities, including Birmingham. Over a period of fifteen months during 1830-1832, seven gangs were arrested in London. At that time, the London resurrectionists were estimated to be about two hundred in number. Some of the most effective resurrectionists were able to exhume, discreetly, about ten bodies during a single night (Wise 2004).

---

[2] *Other common epithets include: "Grave Robbers" "Resurrection Men", "Snatchers", "Grabs", "Lifters", "Body Lifters", "Exhumaters", "Diggum Uppers" "Sack 'em up men", "Resurgem Homo".*

Occasionally turf wars broke out between the gangs *The Birmingham Journal* (November 17th 1827) reported:

"...a gang of resurrection men have recently visited this neighbourhood from London, intending to furnish "subjects" for the winter lectures from the church-yards in this town. An attempt was made this week to remove a corpse that had been interred in St.Martin's church-yard, and every night since a watch has been set upon the grave . We understand that finding their attempts in the town were hazardous, they have laid their scene of action at a few miles distance, though still hovering round Birmingham, as the centre of their attraction."

According to Palmer (2007) and an article entitled *"Black Country Body Snatchers"* in the *Black Country Bugle* of June 18th 2014 by Josephine Jasper, a man named "Brummajem Booth" who lived in Rowley led a gang of resurrectionists who operated throughout the Black Country and transported the bodies to the Birmingham medical school in farm carts concealed under straw and other merchandise[3].

Palmer also includes the following (unsourced) rhyme:

"Here in 1825,

---

[3] *Unfortunately both Mr. Palmer and Ms. Jasper fail to provide the source for their information, so, at best, their accounts must be regarded as local lore.*

The Diggum Uppers

A mon's wuth mower jed than alive
If yow dow believe this dyin' truth
Have a word with Brummagem Booth"

Typically, a member of a grave robbing gang, or his wife, would spend the day loitering in a likely graveyard waiting for a funeral. The spy would even join the mourners in order to take careful note of the appearance of the newly dug grave. Alternatively the gang would be tipped off by informers, (corrupt sextons, grave diggers or undertakers). At night, two members of the gang would appear and, after carefully laying a sheet on the ground, would uncover the head portion of the grave, dumping the loose dirt on the sheet. The body would be pulled from the coffin head first with ropes; the shroud was stuffed back into the grave, the lid replaced and the dirt carefully replaced, (the process took approximately thirty minutes). The body would then be carted off to a medical school and handed over to a   porter, for a price adjusted according to the size and condition of the corpse

However, the grave was not always restored, as in a case of grave robbing at Tettenhall, near Wolverhampton:

"It was discovered, on Friday morning last, that a grave in Tettenhall church-yard had, in the previous night, been disturbed by resurrectionists: the coffin buried therein was wrenched open, and the body it contained appeared to have been taken out, the grave clothes being stripped from it. As the

corpse had been buried nine days, it is supposed to have been found in too advanced a state of putrescence to be worth carrying away: it was therefore relaid in its narrow cell, and slightly covered with soil;. No attempt was made to violate any other grave." (*The Staffordshire Advertiser* 3rd April 1830).

According to Hackwood (1924) the sexton of Wednesbury church known as "*Ode Picks*" was a notorious resurrectionist supplying the Birmingham anatomists. To catch him in the act the local constabulary left an officer posing as a corpse in his care: while he was removing it from the coffin to his wagon, the "corpse" came to life and arrested him. Brought before the magistrates he pleaded:

"Forgive me - I bin a bell-ringer, a psalm-singer at this church for forty 'ear. If yoe'll let me off this time, I'll never rob another stoon, nor touch another boon..."

One resurrectionist who operated in the Black Country was Joseph Grainger of Birmingham.

In November 1827, Grainger was caught by armed guards attempting to steal a cadaver from Aston churchyard (*The Birmingham Journal* 8th December 1827). On the 20th October 1828, Grainger and his accomplice, John Watts, were witnessed by James Murphy in Tipton Graveyard as he was passing: "*It being a clear moonlight night*, [Murphy] *saw two men , one standing on the wall, the other standing on a bench behind the wall and a naked human body laying on the wall*" The Staffordshire Advertiser (24th January 1829) reported. They were apprehended a few hours later; the corpse was identified by Issac Clark as being his son Richard, who had died on the 16th October and had been buried on the 20th. In November 1831 Grainger was arrested, along with his accomplice, Benjamin Sandbrook, following the disinterment of the body of John Fenton who had been buried on October 30th in Smethwick churchyard.

Grainger's accomplice John Watts, (also known as John Pointon), had his own career as a resurrectionist: stealing bodies from churchyards and graveyards across the Black Country, Birmingham, Worcestershire and the Potteries. He was described by *The Worcester Herald* (5th January 1831) as a "*noted rifler of the graves of the dead*".

He was responsible for robbing two graves in Hanley Castle churchyard, Worcestershire. One of which contained Mary Colston of Newbridge Green, Upton upon Severn, who had died at the age of 22; she had been buried on January 11th 1831. The transporting of the bodies to the surgeon in London can be best described as eventful.

Early on the morning of January 21st 1831, Mr. Cale, landlord of The Anchor Inn in Upton, acting as the agent for one of the Worcester coach companies received two wooden crates to be conveyed to London from two men, (one of whom was Watts). The address labels were hammered on by the men using a poker borrowed from Cale and he loaded the crates onto a coach bound for London. However, the following day he heard of the grave robbery in Hanley Castle. Suspecting that the two lifted corpses were in the crates he had sent on, he travelled to London in an attempt to retrieve them. Having obtained the help of a policeman, they tracked down one of the crates, still unopened, to the house of the surgeon John Pocock Holmes[4] in Old Fish Street, Doctors' Commons, in the City of London. The other was eventually found at a police station in Pimlico: having lost its label. Both bodies were reinterred in Hanley Castle. (*The Worcester Journal* 3rd February 1831).

Holmes was forced to defend himself, writing to *The Morning Herald* stating:

"The body taken to my house had been sent by some impudent resurrectionist, who may have known me at the schools, and took the liberty of directing it to my own house, to be left till called for, supposing doubtless, some of his men would fetch the box away, and that I should never know what it contained."

When he was arrested in Birmingham following grave robbery at Hanley and Burslem in the Potteries and at Bilston, Watts had on his person a handwritten

---

[4] *Holmes had invented craniotomy forceps, used in gynaecology, and was the author of "A Treatise on the Employment of Friction and Inhalation in Consumption, Asthma and Other Maladies" (1837).*

letter from a medical student in London to his father, a surgeon *"of considerable practice and eminence"* in Birmingham, implicating him in the grave robbing at Hanley Castle (*The Worcester Herald* 5th February 1831):

"Dear Father- It appears that the man Watts, and his partner here, made a sad mess with the last packages they have sent. This morning two constables from the country called on Mr. Holmes, the surgeon, to whom the parcels were directed, and saw there the first box, which they immediately recognised from the following circumstance. It appears that Watts and the other man went into the house of the constable of the country, and actually borrowed the man's poker to nail on the directions to the box, and thus they (the officers) learned where the parcel was going to. The next day it seems part of the coffin, and a crow bar, were found in the burying ground , and the grave was open. This, of course, led to a suspicion as to the contents of the box; and immediately the constable set off for London, and detected, as I have mentioned, the first box, which contained a young female subject. This they took away with them, and requested Mr. Holmes to be at Guildhall at twelve o'clock: he accordingly went and waited till twenty minutes past, when, as these officers did not make their appearance, he left, and has heard nothing more of the affair, it being now four o'clock. We have heard nothing of the second package, and it is probable it has been either stopped on the road, or at the office in London. Mr. Holmes is a man of a very strong mind; he does not care a farthing about this discovery, which is so far fortunate , but we must alter the direction :- for the future, tell the men to direct to Mr. Smith, at Mr.Saunder's, 18. Devonshire Buildings,

Great Dover Road, London, - They must have managed most wretchedly to go to the constable's house, and to leave the grave open. They must keep out of the way, as the officer knows one of them, and will soon take him into custody. Which it is I do not know, but if they do not mind, they will get taken. I write in haste, therefore excuse this scrawl.

London, Jan.24,1831   Yours, ever, R.D.G."

The difference in accounts possibly results from the medical student, (who was fearful of bring revealed as a customer of Watts), not being aware of the full chain of events.

In March 1831 *The Staffordshire Advertiser* reported that Watts had been found guilty of disinterring and carrying away dead bodies in the Potteries and sentenced to twelve months imprisonment in Stafford gaol and also fined £20. However on 8th October 1831 the newspaper reported he had died in prison of *"pulmonary consumption"* (Tuberculosis).

Workhouses were also a source of cadavers. Partners of resurrectionists would pose as friends or relatives of dying or dead paupers and claim the corpse. Occasionally, corpses would be stolen from family homes where the body had been laid out, prior to burial. One lady, Mrs. Wicks, died on a Monday night and was laid out in her house, with two women watching over her. On the Friday night a man called at the house and convinced the two women to go with him to a nearby public house for a *"comfortable drop"*. When they returned to the house it was found the body had been stolen (*The Staffordshire Advertiser* 14th October 1826).

Despite the risk of imprisonment if caught, the financial rewards of grave robbing were great. A weekly wage for a factory worker in the first quarter of the nineteenth century was approximately 7 shillings (approximately 35 pence today); for a skilled tailor or carpenter: 30 shillings (£1.50) and for a well paid manservant in a wealthy household: 1 guinea a week (£1.05). A cadaver, depending upon freshness and demand, could fetch between 8-20 guineas (between £8.40 and £21.00) (Hurren 2011).

Some cadavers commanded a high premium. Male cadavers were more sought after than female ones, due to their musculature and fresh cadavers and limbs commanded a higher price than ones on the verge of putrefaction. Children's bodies (known as "*smalls*") commanded a high price as did specialty cadavers, (those with congenital disorders or illnesses) (Wise 2004). For example, the surgeon John Hunter paid £500 to procure the body of the Irish giant Charles O'Byrne (1761-1783), whose eight-foot skeleton Hunter wanted for his anatomical museum. This may have been the reason the person buried at the Providence Baptist Chapel in West Bromwich was interred in a mortsafe: it belonged to a young woman (aged 17-25) who in life had suffered from a disfiguring skin and bone disease, possibly metastatic cancer[5]: her body would have fetched a high premium for a resurrectionist (Craddock-Bennett. 2013).

Particular parts of a cadaver, known as "off cuts", such as hair and teeth, could be sold for use by wigmakers and dentists who made the teeth into sets of dentures for wealthy customers.

If a resurrectionist was apprehended, however, it was not necessarily calamitous: surgeons protected their resurrectionists. Sir Astley Paston Cooper was so dependent on the "*London Borough Gang*" for cadavers that he exerted his influence to keep them out of jail on numerous occasions, and, if a member was imprisoned, Cooper paid his family a pension while the breadwinner was serving his term.

An example of this is Joseph Grainger discussed above. Following his arrest in Aston, he received "*an excellent character* [reference] *from some of the surgeons of this town*" (The *Birmingham Journal* 8th December 1827). Documents in the National Archives reveal that following their arrest in 1829, he and his accomplice John Watts were fined £10 each and sentenced to six months imprisonment for stealing the body of Richard Clarke from the burial ground at Tipton. This was despite a petition pleading leniency being sent to

---

[5] *When cancer cells break away from where they first formed and travel through the body to form new tumours in other parts of the body, in this case the skull, femur and spine.*

the home office signed by a number of medical men including William Sands Cox of the Birmingham School of Medicine.

William Sands Cox (1802-1875) was the son of a surgeon. He was educated at King Edward's school, Birmingham, and later studied at Guy's and St.Thomas' Hospitals, London, becoming a surgeon and also a lecturer in anatomy to the Birmingham General Dispensary in 1825. Three years later with the help of Doctors Johnstone, Booth and others, he founded the Birmingham School of Medicine, lecturing there on anatomy and surgery. In 1834, he helped form the provincial Medical and Surgical (now the British Medical) Association and two years later, became a fellow of the Royal Society. During 1840 to 1841, he directed his energies to the foundation of the Queen's Hospital, Birmingham being appointed senior surgeon on its opening.

Following Grainger's, (and Benjamin Sandbrook's), trial in 1832 for stealing the body of John Fenton from Smethwick churchyard a second gaol sentence of six months imprisonment with hard labour and a £10 fine was imposed on Grainger. Sandbrook was given an altogether more lenient sentence of one month's imprisonment with hard labour, even though he had played an equal part in the robbery.

This was due to the view that Grainger was *"addicted to the practice of disinterring dead bodies"* having

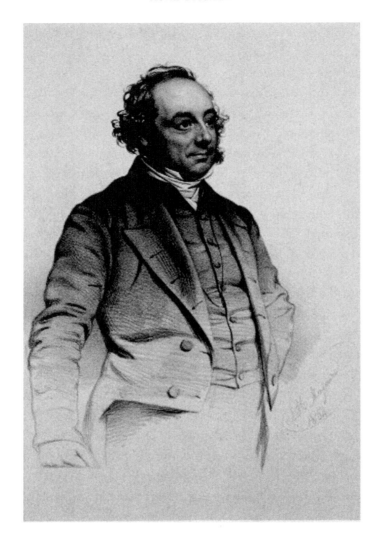

William Sands Cox by T.H. Maguire (1854) (Wellcome)

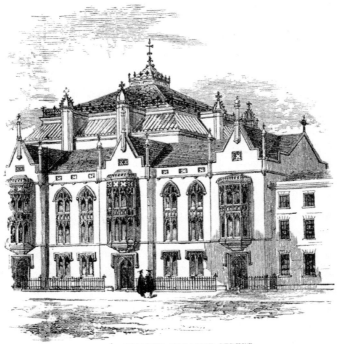

QUEEN'S COLLEGE, PARADISE STREET.

Anatomical School, Queen's College, Paradise Street, Birmingham.

been arrested before and it was believed that Sandbrook had been manipulated by Grainger. On this occasion two petitions were received by the Secretary of State regarding Grainger and Sandbrook requesting leniency: an individual petition by Sands Cox regarding Grainger alone and a petition signed by seven lecturers of the Birmingham School of Medicine regarding both grave robbers.

Sands Cox's petition dated 4th July 1832, requested clemency and reveals that he was supporting Grainger's family throughout his imprisonment:

"The terms of his [Grainger's] sentence is now expired and I most respectfully trust that your Lordship under existing circumstance may be pleased to recommend to his majesty to remit the fine. As lecturer on anatomy at this institution I have compelled my Lord to defray the law expenses and to support his wife and children for the last eight month...when your Lordship considers the evidence on which the individual was convicted and the heavy expenses which have fallen upon me, a young man commencing his profession I am led to anticipate that your Lordship will take the circumstances into your consideration"

A letter from Sir Oswald Moseley, chairman of the quarter sessions for the county of Stafford, shows that he also disagreed with the severity of the punishment: *"I am sorry to observe that the Court of Quarter Sessions exceeded their powers by annexing the punishment of hard labour to the sentences passed upon Grainger and Sandbrook"* and Grainger's fine of £10 was removed.

According to Hackwood (1924), in 1826, Daniel Stone was convicted of disturbing a grave at Upper Gornal. As punishment he was tied to a cart and dragged along the road from Sedgley to Bilston, being whipped as he went.

Thomas Stokes was arrested on the suspicion of having being engaged in grave robbing in the churchyards around Wolverhampton. Described as a *"rogue and a vagabond"* he was sentenced to two months hard labour (*The Birmingham Journal* 23rd February 1828).

The most infamous snatchers, however, were William Burke and William Hare who murdered sixteen people in Edinburgh to supply the surgeon Dr. Robert Knox. When caught in 1828, in return for immunity, Hare turned King's evidence against Burke, who was sentenced to be executed. Following his execution in 1829 Burke was publically dissected in the anatomy theatre of Edinburgh University's Old College, and parts of his skin were used to make wallets, calling card cases and to bind books. His skeleton is on display at the University of Edinburgh's Anatomy Museum (Dudley-Edwards 2014). Dr. Knox, despite public outcry, was never tried for his involvement; although shunned by the medical establishment he continued to teach and write. He died in London in 1862.

Other notorious cases in London in 1831, involved the three resurrectionists: John Bishop,

Thomas Williams and James May who were known as the *"Italian Boy murderers"* or the *"London Burkers"*. In addition to grave robbing they drugged and murdered three people including a 14 year old Italian boy named Carlo Ferrari. The cadavers were sold to anatomists and surgeons from St Bartholomew's Hospital, St Thomas' Hospital and King's College in London. Bishop and Williams were executed and their bodies dissected by surgeons (Wise 2004). Also in London, in the same year, Catherine Walsh of Whitechapel who made her living by selling laces and cotton, was murdered by Elizabeth Ross, who sold the body to surgeons. Ross was hanged for the murder (Donneley 2007).

3) STOPPING THE SNATCHERS

The families of the deceased frequently attempted to deter the resurrectionists, often keeping watch over the fresh grave for two or three weeks until the body had decomposed sufficiently to be useless for dissection. In Scotland, *morthouses* were used, in which corpses were placed until they had decomposed and were then buried.

Watchmen were also employed to guard grave yards and pitched battles occasionally took place between the guards and the resurrectionists, but some guards were open to bribery. *The Birmingham Journal* (4th November 1826) reports the case of a watchman who colluded with a resurrectionist and received 10 shillings for each body to stop him informing. Problems occurred when the watchman was offered a larger sum by a rival resurrectionist, leading to all three being arrested.

When established in 1823 the Bilston Wesleyan Methodist Church graveyard had its own guard to watch over it :

"… it was deemed wise to make a special provision for the protection of the graveyard. Andrew Allen, the caretaker, was employed to watch it, and was furnished with a gun, but was cautioned not to fire, should intruders come, until he had said three times: 'I'm going to shoot'.

'This led to a curious incident. The Trustees had held a prolonged meeting, and had been quite forgotten by Andrew, who had retired to rest for the night, having carefully fastened

the gates. When ready to leave they tried them, and in doing so made some little noise which was quite enough to rouse watchful Andrew. To their surprise his bedroom window casement flew open, and out came his head and gun, and instantly in rapid and angry tones he shouted: 'I'm going to shoot'. The dignified elders found cover with unusually quick movements, and shouted a quiet reassurance to Andrew.

"Andrew had nerves of steel, a quick, salty wit, and a whimsical way of his own, and we cannot forbear another story about him as the graveyard watchman.

"From the window of the old vestry he kept a keen eye on the burial ground, or sat in the late and early hours on a grave, with his heavy stick near, and his gun across his knee. This custom became known in the town, and some revelers at a Swan Bank tavern resolved to frighten him. For a wager one of them borrowed a white sheet from the landlady, and started forth to play the ghost. Appearing at midnight, he remained quiet until St Leonard's chimes were heard marking the hour, when he walked towards Andrew, raising an unearthly moan as he went. Andrew sat quite still as the ghost drew near; presently he stealthily laid aside his gun and reached for his stick, saying: 'I shanna waste powder on ghoses – I'll try the stick,' and before the intruder was aware of his movements he was soundly rapping his head and shoulders with his cudgel, and had snatched off the sheet and torn it into many pieces, saying: 'I'll gie thee playing ghoses on me.' (Freeman 1923 p.137-8).

A similar incident occurred in St. Phillip's graveyard, Birmingham in April 1830 when a woman named Marshall and some friends had been standing guard at night over the grave of her infant to protect it from resurrectionists. A mischievous youth disguised himself as a ghost to scare the guards. However, when he appeared, the mother immediately seized the ghost, and despite his threats, held him secure until a watchman arrived and took him to the lock up (*The Birmingham Journal* 8th May 1830).

Booby traps were also utilised. One grieving father filled his child's coffin with gunpowder and fused it so that it would explode if disturbed. Another booby trap was the cemetery gun. These guns were set up at the foot of a grave, with three tripwires strung in an arc around its position. Those who stumbled upon one in the dark may have found themselves in a grave of their own, or seriously wounded. They were outlawed in 1827, (Guttmacher 1935; Orly 1999).

Others sought to make the graves of their loved ones secure against the resurrectionists by using coffins made of iron or mortsafes, such as the one found at West Bromwich.

The mortsafe was invented around 1816. These were iron or iron and stone devices of great weight, in different designs. Often they were complex, heavy contraptions of rods and plates, padlocked together. A plate was placed over the coffin and rods with heads were pushed through holes in it. These rods were kept in place by locking a second plate over the first to form extremely heavy protection. It could only be removed by two people with keys. The safes were placed over the coffins for about six weeks, then removed for further use when the body inside was sufficiently decomposed. Sometimes a church bought them and hired them out. Societies were also formed to purchase them and control their use, with annual membership fees, and charges made to non-members.

Other examples of attempts to deter the resurrectionists found in the West Bromwich Providence chapel graveyard included a brick grave in which a corpse had been buried in two coffins: the outer coffin secured with thick timber and iron; a thick pine plank, longer than the coffin, placed on top of a coffin and the ends recessed into the ends of the grave and iron bars laid across a coffin at chest and knee level. (Craddock-Bennett 2013).

Other mortsafes utilised iron bars and slabs of stone.

The Staffordshire Advertiser (7th February 1829) carried an advertisement for the *"Schofield Safety Tomb"* designed to *"frustrate all the efforts of Resurrection men...it will not only prevent resurrectionists from succeeding in their nefarious objects, but will also punish them for their attempt...There are also such other contrivances within, (which is not prudent to describe,) that if any person have the temerity to attempt an entrance after dark, or after the vault is secured, he must suffer the consequences of it"*. Unfortunately the advertisement fails to divulge what the consequences would be.

Aris's Birmingham Gazette advertised extra secure coffins:

"In consequence of the alarming reports that are in

circulation in this town and its vicinity of bodies being stolen from Church and Chapel Yards, the Public are respectfully informed, that they may be supplied with WOODEN COFFINS, of which the maker will defy any possibility of their being re-opened by the Resurrection Men, at a trifling extra expense of a common coffin.

"Apply to W. Faulconbridge and Co, Packing Box and Case-makers, Staniforth-street, near the Black Boy" (9th February 1829).

Unfortunately, such protection was often only available to those who could afford it. However, other methods were suggested:

"RESURRECTIONISTS. - A clergyman suggests the following plan, which he has adopted in his own church-yard, and has also recommended it to several of his friends: - Cover the coffin with earth, until within half a yard or more (as circumstances may admit), of the surface of the ground; then lower down the top stone which usually covers the grave, and afterwards let the whole be perfectly filled up, and remain so for about half a year or more, or if the friends of the deceased can afford it, a stone nearly the size of the grave may be gently let down into the grave, after each interment, having previously thrown about a half foot of earth over the coffin" (*The Birmingham Journal* 28th March 1829).

The Birmingham Journal also recommended that as the grave was being filled, alternate layers of straw or shavings be laid down *"...so that the insertion of a spade for the purpose of opening the grave is considerably checked, and the labour of the resurrectionist greatly augmented, if not rendered entirely abortive."* (16th February 1828).

35

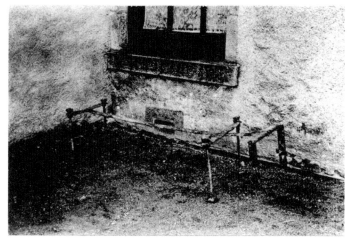

*Above: A mort-safe from Oyne, Aberdeenshire similar to
the one found at the providence chapel West Bromwich
(Wellcome).*
*Below: Mortsafe St. Nicholas' Church, Loxley, Warwickshire
(Author)*

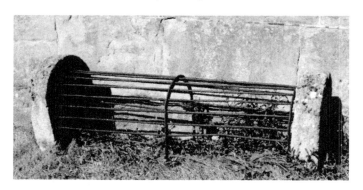

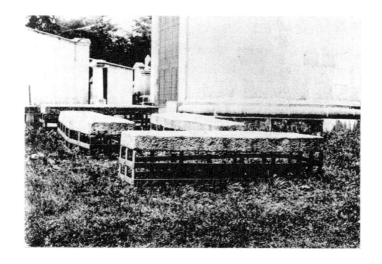

Mortsafes in Cluny graveyard, Aberdeenshire (Wellcome)

4) THE ANATOMY ACT

The trade in cadavers had reached massive proportions. More than once large shipments of bodies from the public graveyards in Ireland and other countries packed in piano cases and kegs were left unclaimed on the docks of Liverpool and London: which did not fail to attract the attention of the authorities (Guttmacher 1935). For example, the *Wolverhampton Chronicle and Staffordshire Advertiser* (20th January 1830) reported that *"A vessel recently sailed from Ostend, with a cargo of dead bodies, intended for the London resurrectionists"*. Also, faced with public outrage over the cases of Burke and Hare, "The London Burkers" and Elizabeth Ross, the government brought the trade of the resurrectionists to a halt by introducing the Anatomy Act in 1832. Under the Act only physicians and surgeons had legal access to, (i.e. they could legitimately purchase), corpses which were unclaimed after death in prisons, hospitals, asylums and workhouses providing no relatives of the deceased objected. The Act also revoked the legislation permitting the dissection of murderers (Hurren 2011).

However, the Act was open to abuse.

According to Ruth Richardson (2001): *"What had for generations been a feared and hated punishment for murder became one for poverty."* (p.270-71). While relatives of the paupers who had died in such institutions could object to the bodies of their dear ones being dissected: they had to object within seven days of the death and provide the money to pay for a coffin and churchyard burial. If they couldn't afford this, then the remains could - quite legitimately within the regulations of the Anatomy Act - be sent to a teaching hospital for dissection in return for a fee which contributed to the income of the Workhouse. Some unscrupulous workhouse keepers would post notices of deaths in such long, convoluted language that those paupers who had only a basic grasp of reading would be unable to understand that one of their relatives had died and be unable to protest, (Richardson 2001, Hurren 2011).

On 11th June 1844, a debate in the House of Commons confirmed that between 1839 and 1841, the bodies of some three hundred paupers had been dissected - quite legitimately - under the provisions of the Anatomy Act. It was also observed that not all workhouse masters were putting the fee paid for a corpse into the workhouse funds but were entering the death into the union's Dead-Book and then pocketing the fee for themselves. However, it was decided this was a matter for individual workhouse unions to address and not a suitable matter for Parliament to handle. It was also stated that when corpses and body parts were no longer required in one place, they were not being buried with the appropriate dignity and rites, but sold on, at a profit, to other hospitals and that lecturers were often adding to their own incomes through this practice. Once more Parliament refused to address the issue saying it was up to individual medical schools to control this. The plea of some Parliamentarians to set up a commission to investigate these matters fell upon deaf ears and their motion was soundly defeated.

Such abuses were occurring in the workhouses of the Black Country.

In 1873, the governors of the West Bromwich Union Workhouse declared that paupers in need of medical care had to come into the workhouse. However, if they died and could not afford a pauper funeral then their body would be treated as unclaimed and sold for a small fee to Queen's College Anatomical School in Birmingham. In this way their welfare debt to society would be repaid (Hurren 2011). Mr. Hampton, a guardian of the Union, exposed the practice in *The Birmingham Daily Post* of 13th March 1877. It was reported that at a meeting of the Union Guardians, Mr. Hampton alleged, supported by Mr. Ward, (another guardian), that bodies taken from the workhouse for dissection were being treated disrespectfully: bodies were being taken away naked without a shroud in a covered wagon, the heads being knocked as they were being thrown into the wagon. Both men demanded to know how the bodies of paupers were being sent to the anatomy school and what burial rites were they given?

Mr. Gilpin, the workhouse master denied the allegations:

"[A] *body to which* [they] *referred was properly dressed, put in a shroud and removed in a shell to the Dead-House. It was lifted into the coffin in the shroud, and was taken away to Birmingham in the coffin. He thought it was not necessary to have the body disturbed* [i.e. exhumed to ensure this was the case]. *He did not see the conveyance but was under the impression that it was a proper hearse"* (*The Birmingham Daily Post* 13th March 1877).

The chairman emphasised that the journey of each pauper corpse from West Bromwich Union workhouse to the anatomy school at Birmingham appeared to be a *"Pauper funeral"*. It is interesting to note that the guardians did not refer to these procedures as *"Anatomy funerals"* which, while being far more accurate, would have caused outcry among the locals due to the stigma attached, especially as in a pauper funeral and burial the body would be buried within the parish boundaries. The transportation of the corpses was done at night to avoid any bad publicity, but with the cat having been released from the bag, the chairman was quick to reassure that the final burial of the remains was either in consecrated ground, if a Christian, or in a burial ground appropriate to the religious denomination to which the person belonged when alive (i.e. Roman Catholic, Methodist, Baptist, Quaker, etc.). However, he avoided giving details of where each corpse was buried, the state of the body when buried and whether the body had been treated with dignity after dissection.

In the winter of 1889 James Clarke, a pauper,

died in the Walsall Union Workhouse. The clerk of the workhouse noted that Clarke was a tramp with no relations and his corpse was sold to Queen's College Anatomical School, Birmingham, where it was dissected and dismembered by the Chair of Anatomy, Professor Bertram C.A.Windle. Finished with, the remains were placed in a very basic coffin shell known as a "*deal box*" and buried on 31st January 1890 in common ground at Witton cemetery, Birmingham, in a multiple grave. The common ground had been allocated to the anatomical school by the City authorities to bury dissected cadavers, some insufficient to fill a deal box.

A fortnight later, James Clarke's widow arrived at the workhouse. She was told by the workhouse master that her husband was dead and the body had been removed. She left under the impression that her husband had received a pauper burial and been buried within the parish boundaries. A week later, Clarke's daughter, Mrs. Margaret Longmine (neé Clarke) called at the workhouse. She had been estranged from her father for some time and had been searching for him unaware he was destitute. When told he had died and been given a pauper's burial she asked to see the grave – a request that alarmed the workhouse master. She insisted she should be shown his grave because she wished to give her father a proper headstone.

The master was in a quandary: he couldn't show her the grave without betraying the fact her father's body was in Birmingham and not in a Walsall parish grave. The Walsall guardians had not advertised the fact they had agreed to be suppliers to the anatomy trade for fear of public outcry. Fearing – and hoping to avoid – public exposure, the master wrote to Professor Windle outlining Mrs. Longmine's case: "*When they* [Mrs.Longmine and her husband] *write to me again, as they probably will do, I should inform them of the fact, which they do not at present seem to have grasped that their father's body has been submitted to complete dissection and that the remaining fragments have been duly buried*" (p.70 Hurren 2011).

Professor Windle referred the case to the Inspectors at the Anatomy Inspectorate: the government department which governed the use of bodies by anatomy schools. The Inspectorate replied that both men had acted correctly under the strict letter of the law. They also informed them that as Clarke's widow, and not her daughter, had first legal claim on the body they could refer any further queries to the Inspectorate in London. While the Inspectorate would give them legal advice, the two men should suppress any scandal. Nor could they elaborate regarding the difference between a "*pauper burial*" and an "*anatomy burial*" in print: the matter was to be kept confidential (Huron 2011).

A memorandum was issued on the 28th November 1889 and attached to the Anatomy Inspectorate file on James Clarke: it reminded everyone concerned that the work of the Anatomical schools was covered by the Official Secrets Act of 1889 (Huron 2011). Any negative publicity would be detrimental and legislation decreed there could be no further official discussion. Evidence that the Victorian government was concerned enough to suppress knowledge of the anatomy trade. Even Professor Windle admitted it was better that the bereaved did not understand what occurred (Hurren 2011).

A skeleton of a young male was uncovered, at the West Bromwich Providence Chapel that bore the signs of having undergone an autopsy: the skull had been sawn horizontally across the forehead and the vertebrae cut through, suggesting the spinal cord had been removed (Craddock-Bennett. 2013). Were these the remains of someone who died in a Birmingham hospital and whose body was claimed by his family for a private burial in their local churchyard, yet, unbeknownst to them, had been subject to dissection?

Not all bodies were transported to Queen's College in Birmingham. Professor Arthur Thompson purchased, on behalf of the Oxford University Anatomical School, two bodies in 1886, and two in 1887, from the Wolverhampton Workhouse, (on the same trip in 1886 he also brought three from Birmingham) (Hurren 2011).

.

.

5) IT DOESN'T HAPPEN TODAY...

The 1832 Anatomy Act was not repealed until the introduction of the 1984 Anatomy Act which was introduced to address the issue of organ transplants. This was superseded by the Human Tissue Act 2004 which made it illegal to remove, store or use human tissue without appropriate consent.

The Human Tissue Act arose from the scandals in the 1980's and 1990's at Alder Hey Children's Hospital, Liverpool, (HMSO 2001a) and Bristol Royal Infirmary (HMSO 2001b) in which both hospitals were found guilty of keeping organs from dead children without the consent of parents. However, in 2012 it was revealed that a number of police forces in the United Kingdom had stored the body parts of hundreds of murder victims without the knowledge of their relatives (Daily Telegraph 2012).

Further, in 2015, it was revealed that the Biological Research Centre, Arizona, United States, which brokered the donation of human bodies for medical research had been selling the bodies to a United States Army research project for use in blast testing. The owner Stephen Gore was sentenced to between two and a half years to seven years in prison for mishandling the donations

REFERENCES

Anonymous Ballard (c.1820) *Not A Trap Was Heard.* Printed by Jackson & Son, Printers, 21, Moor-street, Birmingham.

Burch, D. (2007). *Digging Up the Dead: Uncovering the Life and Times of an Extraordinary Surgeon. Vintage.*

Craddock-Bennett, L. (2013), 'Providence Chapel and burial ground, Sandwell, West Bromwich', *Post-Medieval Archaeology. 47*:2, 382–6.

Daily Telegraph (21 May 2012*) Body parts of hundreds of murder victims stored by police for decades.*

Donnely. P. (2007) *Essex Murders.* Wharncliffe Books

Dudley-Edwards, O. (2014) *Burke and Hare.* Birlinn Ltd.

Frank,J.B. (1976) Body Snatching: A Grave Medical Problem. *The Yale Journal Of Biology And Medicine 49*, 399-410.

Freeman, J. (1931) *Black Country Stories and Sketches.* James Wilkes: Bilston.

Guttmacher, A. F., *(1935)* Bootlegging bodies. A history of body-snatching. *Bulletin of the Society of Medical History. 4, 353-412.*

Hackwood F.W. (1924) *Staffordshire Customs, Superstitions and Folklore.* E.P.Publishing: Yorkshire.

Her Majesty's Stationary Office (2001a) *The Royal Liverpool Children's Inquiry Report.*

-- -- (2001b) *The report of the public inquiry into children's heart surgery at the Bristol Royal Infirmary 1984-*

1995: learning from Bristol.

Hurren, E. (2011) *Dying for Victorian Medicine: English Anatomy and its Trade in the Dead Poor, c.1834 – 1929* . Palgrave MacMillan

Jasper, J. (2014) *"Black Country Body Snatchers" The Black Country Bugle June 18th* .

Moore, W. (2006) *The Knife Man: Blood, Body-snatching and the Birth of Modern Surgery*. Bantam.

National Archives. *Individual petition (William Sands Cox) and 1 collective petition (7 lecturers of the Birmingham School of Medicine and Surgery) on behalf of Joseph Grainger convicted with Benjamin Sandbrook at Stafford Quarter Sessions in January 1832 for stealing the dead body of John Fenton from a church yard in Smethwick on 31 October 1831.*

Olry, R. (1999) Body Snatchers: the Hidden Side of the History of Anatomy. *J Int Soc Plastination 14 (2)*: 6-9

Palmer, R. (2007) *The Folklore of the Black Country.* Logaston Press.

Quigley, C. (2012)_*Dissection on Display: Cadavers, Anatomists and Public Spectacle*. McFarland & Co

Richardson, R. (2001) *Death, dissection and the destitute*. London, Phoenix Press.

Wise, S (2004) *The Italian Boy: Murder and Grave-robbery in 1830s London*. Johnathon Cape Ltd.

Young, S. (1890) *Annals of the Barber Surgeons.* Appendix C. London: Blades East & Blades, 1890.

Printed in Great Britain
by Amazon

37779136R10036